The Price Effects of Hospital Mergers:
A Case Study of the Sutter-Summit Transaction

I.   Introduction

The antitrust agencies regularly forecast whether prospective mergers are likely to be anticompetitive. Assessment of their success in this mission is complicated by two selection problems. First, it is difficult to analyze whether a blocked merger would have benefited consumers, since no post-merger activity is ever observed. Similarly, since the antitrust authorities try to prevent (or modify) the most egregious transactions, relatively few plausibly anticompetitive mergers are actually completed. For these reasons, evidence regarding the competitive effects of consummated mergers is relatively scarce (Vita and Sacher, 2001). This shortcoming limits evaluation of whether prospective merger analysis provides a reliable estimate of a transaction's future competitive impact.

To help fill this void, we conduct a retrospective study of a consummated hospital merger. In this transaction, Sutter, a network of non-profit hospitals, acquired Summit, a non-profit hospital located in Oakland, California. This combined Summit with Sutter's Alta Bates hospital in Berkeley, California. The two hospitals were approximately 2½ miles apart. The San Francisco Bay Area contained many other hospitals that offered a similar range of services, but which were located farther away. A central issue raised by the Sutter-Summit transaction was whether travel costs were low enough such that these hospitals were a sufficient constraint on the merging parties to prevent an anticompetitive price increase.

Although the Federal Trade Commission (FTC) took no action in this matter, the California Attorney General unsuccessfully tried to block it. Since an antitrust suit was brought, but did not ultimately prevail, this transaction provides a case study of a merger that was consummated despite raising antitrust concern. This allows us to analyze whether antitrust enforcement was too lax for what might be viewed as a marginal case, since the FTC and the

California Attorney General pursued different enforcement actions.[1] The success of both the antitrust agencies and the courts in analyzing such mergers is of great policy importance for two reasons. First, even a relatively minor change in antitrust enforcement potentially affects mergers that are "close calls." Second, and perhaps more importantly, changes in enforcement policy influence which transactions are ever attempted in the first place.

Our analysis focuses on a fundamental question regarding the Sutter-Summit transaction: how does each hospital's price adjust after the merger, and is this price change sufficiently unusual that it can be reasonably attributed to the transaction? We are able to answer this question due to the availability of a particularly rich data source: detailed claims data from the merging hospitals and three large health insurers.[2] We find that Summit charged significantly less than Alta Bates did prior to the transaction, but post-merger the two prices converged. Although Alta Bates' post-merger price change is similar to the price change for other hospitals, Summit's price increase is one of the largest of any comparable hospital in California. The empirical evidence indicates that, for this transaction, the merger of a higher priced hospital with a lower priced competitor produced two higher priced hospitals (section II discusses why the merger led to a price increase at Summit, but not Alta Bates).

The key implication of our results is that this transaction may have been anticompetitive.[3] Our findings therefore support the FTC's 2002 decision, made subsequent to the Sutter-Summit

---

[1] The San Francisco Chronicle reported, "Legal sources said the FTC ducked the case because the federal courts have been reluctant to block any hospital mergers, particularly those in urban areas served by many hospitals." ("Proposed Hospital Merger Goes on Trial." *San Francisco Chronicle*, October 26, 1999).

[2] The data was obtained through the FTC's program of hospital merger retrospectives. A 2002 speech by former FTC Chairman Timothy Muris provides additional details on this program ("Everything Old is New Again: Health Care and Competition in the 21st Century." Prepared Remarks of Timothy J. Muris before the 7th Annual Competition in Health Care Forum, November 7, 2002).

[3] A full determination of whether antitrust enforcement was appropriate in this matter requires analysis of two additional issues that are beyond the scope of this study. First, the merger's impact on hospital quality would have to be considered. Second, Summit may have been a "failing firm." A highly contested issue in the Sutter-Summit preliminary injunction trial, the judge ultimately concluded that the defendants had successfully established a failing firm defense. California v. Sutter Health System, 130 F. Supp. 2d at 1137 (N.D. California, 2001). It may have been better to allow the merger if blocking it would have resulted in Summit leaving the market altogether.

transaction, to form a merger litigation task force with the purpose of "reinvigorating the Commission's hospital merger program."[4]

Our findings highlight two other important issues. First, they do not support the proposition that mergers involving non-profit hospitals are not of antitrust concern, as has previously been suggested (see section II). We find a substantial price increase even though the merging parties were both non-profits. Second, our findings call into question the applicability to hospital mergers of the Elzinga-Hogarty (1973 and 1978) method for delineating the geographic market in which to analyze a transaction. Both sides relied upon this approach in the Sutter-Summit preliminary injunction trial. In this method, the geographic market is constructed so that it has limited patient inflow and outflow. As previous research shows, however, substantial patient flows across two geographic areas is insufficient to conclude that competition from hospitals in one area will prevent a post-merger price increase in the other. This is confirmed in our results.

The layout of the paper is as follows. Section II presents background information and discusses related literature. Econometric issues are detailed in section III. Section IV describes the data. Section V presents results. Section VI concludes.

II.   Merger Background and Related Literature

The Sutter-Summit transaction attracted antitrust attention from both the FTC and the California Attorney General due to the overlap between Summit and Sutter's Alta Bates hospital, located approximately 2½ miles away in Berkeley, California. While the FTC did not take enforcement action, on August 11, 1999 the California Attorney General filed a complaint in federal court to block the transaction. The motion for a preliminary injunction was denied on

---

[4] "Federal Trade Commission Announces Formation of Merger Litigation Task Force." FTC press release, August 28, 2002.

December 27, 1999, and the two hospitals merged a few hours later. Below, we highlight the key issues raised by the Sutter-Summit transaction.

Market Definition

Market definition plays a major role in merger analysis. This entails delineation of both a product and a geographic market within which the competitive effect of a proposed merger is analyzed.[5] In cases involving hospital mergers, the courts generally support a product market of acute inpatient care (Sacher and Silvia, 1998; Gaynor and Vogt, 1999). For other services, such as outpatient surgery, hospitals are assumed to have relatively little market power since they face significant competition from non-hospital sources.[6] In the preliminary injunction trial, both sides agreed that acute inpatient care comprised the relevant product market. We follow precedent and similarly focus our analysis on this set of services.

Geographic market definition was a central point of contention in the preliminary injunction trial. This was such a crucial issue because more than twenty hospitals were located either in San Francisco or in the area to the east known as the East Bay.[7] Many of these hospitals provided a wide range of services similar to those available at Summit and Alta Bates. If they were close substitutes for Summit and Alta Bates then the proposed transaction likely would not pose a competitive problem.

The substitutability of these hospitals may be limited by their geographic dispersion across a large metropolitan region. The California Attorney General argued that, among other factors, substantial commuting times across the San Francisco Bay Area made the relevant geographic area in which to analyze the transaction a much smaller region known as the "Inner

---

[5] The courts have generally followed the analytic framework detailed in the FTC and DOJ's Horizontal Merger Guidelines. Market definition is a key step in this analysis.

[6] See, for example, Judge Posner's decision in Hospital Corporation of America v. Federal Trade Commission, 807 F.2d 1381 (7th Circuit, 1986).

[7] California v. Sutter Health System, 130 F. Supp. 2d at 1112 (N.D. California, 2001).

East Bay."[8] This proposed geographic market excluded numerous hospitals in the broader metropolitan area, implying that Summit and Alta Bates would have a combined market share of nearly 50%.[9]

In the preliminary injunction trial, each side employed Elzinga-Hogarty (1973 and 1978) analysis either to defend a preferred geographic market, or to construct a geographic market in the first place. This methodology uses patient flow data to determine geographic boundaries. The relevant market is expanded until "most" patients who reside in that region choose to receive care there, and until "most" patients outside the area do not travel into the proposed geographic market to seek hospital services.[10,11] That is, the geographic market is constructed so that it has limited patient inflow and outflow.

The Elzinga-Hogarty method for delineating the geographic market has been widely critiqued.[12] Depending on the homogeneity of the hospitals involved and the level of travel costs, the Elzinga-Hogarty approach can either overstate or understate the willingness of consumers to substitute between hospitals (Werden, 1981 and 1990). Capps et al. (2001) explain how the presence of a significant number of individuals with low travel costs may say little about the substitution patterns of those who face higher travel costs.

---

[8] The Inner East Bay encompasses the area "between the San Francisco Bay on the west and the Caldecott Tunnel on the east, and running from the Carquinez Strait in the north to Union City in the south." California v. Sutter Health System, 130 F. Supp. 2d at 1121 (N.D. California, 2001).

[9] "Proposed Hospital Merger Goes on Trial." *San Francisco Chronicle*, October 26, 1999.

[10] In practice, "most" is usually between 75% and 90% (Elzinga and Hogarty, 1973 and 1978).

[11] Each side applied the Elzinga-Hogarty method in a different manner. The plaintiff's expert expanded the market by sequentially adding zip codes where Summit and Alta Bates had the largest *share* of patients. In contrast, the defendant's expert sequentially added zip codes from which Summit and Alta Bates drew the largest *number* of patients.

[12] In a recent trial, Kenneth Elzinga testified on behalf of the FTC that the Elzinga-Hogarty approach is not an appropriate method for delineating the geographic market in hospital mergers. Evanston Northwestern Healthcare Corp., FTC Docket No. 9315, Initial Decision (Oct. 20, 2005).

Nonetheless, based in part on each side's Elzinga-Hogarty analysis, the judge rejected the plaintiff's proposed Inner East Bay geographic market. The judge noted that 15% of patients living in that area went to hospitals located elsewhere, and that 15% of those going to hospitals in the Inner East Bay lived outside the area.[13] Support for a wider market implies that the judge believed Summit and Alta Bates faced competition from numerous other hospitals, and suggested a low perceived likelihood that the proposed transaction would be anticompetitive.[14]

A virtue of a retrospective study is that it does not require delineation of the relevant geographic market. Rather, we simply analyze each hospital's post-merger price change. This allows independent assessment of the Elzinga-Hogarty approach. If the methodology was appropriate in this matter, then the significant patient inflows and outflows reported above suggest the transaction was unlikely to be anticompetitive.[15] This paper investigates whether this was indeed the case.

Competitive Effects

Researchers have developed a number of empirical methods for predicting the competitive effect of hospital mergers (Town and Vistnes, 2001; Capps et al., 2003; Gaynor and Vogt, 2003).[16] The commonality across these approaches is that the competitive impact of a

---

[13] California v. Sutter Health System, 130 F. Supp. 2d at 1124 (N.D. California, 2001).

[14] The judge also discussed the incentive of Managed Care Organizations and Independent Practice Associations to steer patients towards low-cost providers. Diversion of patients to other hospitals would constrain the merging parties' ability to enact a post-merger price increase. California v. Sutter Health System, 130 F. Supp. 2d at 1129 (N.D. California, 2001).

[15] What constitutes "significant" patient flow is inherently subjective. While the judge in the preliminary injunction trial believed the level of patient flow between the Inner East Bay and the greater metropolitan area was substantial, the California Attorney General argued otherwise based on the same evidence.

[16] After delineation of the relevant product and geographic market, the next step typically taken in merger analysis is to consider the competitive impact of the transaction within the delineated market. The judge in the Sutter-Summit preliminary injunction trial concluded that the California Attorney General had failed to delineate a proper market. Since market definition is a necessary predicate to the competitive effects analysis, the judge's decision contains relatively little discussion of competitive effects.

merger depends on the degree to which patients view the merging parties as substitutes.[17] Broadly speaking, consumer preferences regarding hospital choice can be decomposed into three factors: i) the breadth of services offered; ii) geographic location; and iii) hospital quality. Breadth of services is a key consideration since consumers can choose between only those hospitals that offer the particular service they require. From among those hospitals, consumers presumably prefer higher quality care provided in a convenient location (e.g., near their home).

Summit and Alta Bates were close substitutes with respect to breadth of services offered. Both offered a wide range of hospital services. Furthermore, they were located only 2½ miles apart, a feature that enhances substitutability for those who prefer receiving hospital care in the Oakland-Berkeley area. The greatest apparent difference between the two was each hospital's reputation for quality. Alta Bates was viewed as the higher quality institution.[18]

Its inferior reputation may explain why Summit attracted far fewer commercial patients than Alta Bates even though it had lower prices (giving health insurers an incentive to steer patients to Summit). State discharge data from 1999 reveals that of the patients admitted to the six hospitals located in the immediate vicinity of Oakland-Berkeley, Alta Bates accounted for 42% of commercial admissions, whereas Summit accounted for only 15%.[19]

An alternative means of quantifying this difference is to calculate each hospital's share of admissions using a method developed by Capps and Dranove (2004). A given hospital's admission share is calculated separately for each zip code, and then a weighted average is taken

---

[17] For ease of exposition, we refer to patients as being the one who chooses a hospital. We recognize that, in practice, this decision is jointly determined by the patient, his doctor, and the health insurer (who may offer incentives to steer patients to a particular hospital).

[18] The judge's decision in the preliminary injunction trial notes that Alta Bates is a "comprehensive community hospital that enjoys a reputation for quality health care services." In contrast, when describing Summit the judge did not highlight the quality of the hospital's services. California v. Sutter Health System, 130 F. Supp. 2d at 1112 (N.D. California, 2001).

[19] In contrast, Summit accounted for 32% of non-commercial admissions, compared to only 20% for Alta Bates.

based on the fraction of the hospital's admissions that come from each zip code.[20] This provides a market share measure that does not require delineation of a particular geographic market (which as detailed above, was highly contested).

For Alta Bates, this computation reveals that, on average, it accounted for 44% of commercial admissions in the zip codes from which it drew patients, while Summit had an 11% share of admissions. In contrast, Summit had an average admission share of 14% across the zip codes from which it drew patients, while Alta Bates had a 31% share. Although Alta Bates was Summit's largest competitor, Summit was a relatively small provider of hospital services to commercial patients. In antitrust matters, the argument is often raised that a larger producer is, all else equal, a greater price constraint on a smaller rival than the reverse.[21] If this were the case here, the implication is that the Sutter-Summit transaction would have led to a much larger price increase for Summit than for Alta Bates. Our empirical analysis tests whether this happened.

Despite this asymmetry between Summit and Alta Bates, the two hospitals are more similar to each other than to the four other hospitals located in the immediate vicinity of Oakland-Berkeley:

i) Kaiser hospital in Oakland offered a comparable range of services to Summit and Alta Bates. However, it competed with other hospitals only indirectly since Kaiser is a vertically integrated health care provider that serves patients covered by its health plans. As such, health insurers could not choose Kaiser Oakland as an alternative to Summit and Alta Bates when forming their hospital networks.

ii) Alameda County Medical Center was the largest hospital in the East Bay region, but performed a somewhat narrower range of services compared to Summit and Alta Bates. It had a

---

[20] To control for differences in the services offered at each hospital, Capps and Dranove (2004) calculate market shares for each combination of zip code and major diagnostic category. As a robustness check, we repeated the analysis in this manner and obtained similar results.

[21] See, for example, Inova Health System Foundation and Prince William Health System, Inc., FTC Docket No. 9326, Administrative Complaint (May 8, 2008). The complaint alleges that competition between the two hospitals particularly constrains prices at the smaller hospital.

reputation for being unattractive to commercial patients, and instead primarily served indigent and low-income residents of Alameda County. State discharge data from 1999 reveal that less than 3% of the hospital's admissions were covered by commercial health plans, with the majority of admissions accounted for by either Medicaid or county indigent care programs.[22]

iii) Children's hospital provided only pediatric care.

iv) Alameda hospital was a small community hospital that offered a narrow range of services.

Due to these differences with the four other hospitals located in the immediate area, Summit and Alta Bates were arguably each other's closest substitute in the Oakland-Berkeley area. The key question, therefore, is whether consumers were willing to substitute to hospitals in the San Francisco Bay Area that offered similar services, but which were located farther away. If travel costs were sufficiently low then those living in Oakland-Berkeley would have numerous other practical alternatives in the greater metropolitan area, limiting the merging parties' ability to raise price post-merger. In this retrospective study, we analyze whether the merger led to higher prices. If so, that would suggest consumers were unwilling to incur substantial travel costs to avoid a price increase.

Non-Profit Status

The Sutter-Summit transaction involved the merger of non-profit hospitals. In previous cases, the courts have appeared willing to accept that non-profit hospital mergers pose less risk to competition (Gaynor and Vogt, 1999).[23] One rationale for this belief is that non-profit hospitals may act in the best interests of the community (Lynk, 1995). For example, non-profit hospitals

---

[22] In comparison, 19% and 52% of Summit and Alta Bates' admissions were of commercial patients, respectively.

[23] Notably, however, the judge rejected this argument in a recent trial involving a consummated hospital merger. Evanston Northwestern Healthcare Corp., FTC Docket No. 9315, Initial Decision (Oct. 20, 2005).

may behave like a consumer cooperative, setting price to maximize the welfare of those in the surrounding area. In this case, a hospital merger offers little incentive to raise price.

Other assumptions regarding a hospital's utility function have different competitive implications (Harrison and Lybecker, 2005). For instance, a hospital's objective might be to maximize the prestige of those who run it (Newhouse, 1970). Alternatively, a hospital may wish to maximize the charitable care it provides. If those receiving charity care are a distinct group from those being charged for care, then a non-profit would set the same price as a for-profit hospital (since profit maximization coincides with charity care maximization). Given the wide range of possible assumptions regarding the objective function of non-profit hospitals, determining whether non-profit hospital mergers have a different likelihood of being anticompetitive is ultimately an empirical question.

A number of empirical studies address this issue (Lynk, 1995; Simpson and Shin, 1998; Dranove and Ludwick, 1999; Keeler et al., 1999; Lynk and Neumann, 1999; Vita and Sacher, 2001). Gaynor and Vogt (1999) find mixed results in their survey of the literature, with the post-merger price increase of non-profit hospitals ranging from essentially zero to effects as large as 17%.[24] As Gaynor and Vogt point out, however, differences in methodology and data complicate making comparisons between them. Given the heterogeneity of the obtained results, the antitrust implications of non-profit status remain unresolved.

Previous Hospital Merger Studies

A number of papers analyze the competitive effects of hospital mergers. The most relevant to this paper are those that employ an event study methodology.[25] For example, Vita

---

[24] With the exception of Vita and Sacher, these papers analyze changes in market concentration. Gaynor and Vogt therefore report the predicted price change from a merger within a market comprised of five identically sized hospitals.

[25] Gaynor and Vogt (1999) and Vita and Sacher (2001) discuss earlier studies which employ a Structure-Conduct-Performance approach.

and Sacher (2001) use a "difference in difference" estimator that compares the post-transaction price change of the merging hospitals to a control group. Other studies look at price effects across multiple mergers, such as Conner et al. (1998) and Krishnan (2001).[26]

This study differs from those preceding it in a number of important dimensions. First, it employs a very rich dataset. Rather than relying on aggregate-level data, where it is difficult to control for heterogeneity across patients, we employ highly detailed claims-level data. Our data reports transaction prices, rather than the list prices often employed in previous research. Further, the large number of hospitals in our dataset allows us to compare the merging parties' post-merger price change to the entire distribution of price changes for the control group hospitals. Doing so explicitly recognizes the substantial price change heterogeneity that exists even across hospitals with similar observable characteristics. As discussed in the following section, this allows us to distinguish merger effects from inter-hospital differences that would arise even in the absence of the transaction.

III.   Model Specification

This section details the estimation approach we employ to analyze the impact of the Sutter-Summit transaction on prices at Summit and Alta Bates. We follow the commonly used approach of measuring the post-merger price change relative to the price change for a control group that did not undergo merger (e.g., Vita and Sacher, 2001; Taylor and Hosken, 2007). Since California is a large state containing many hospitals, we are able to employ a two-stage estimation approach that constructs the standard error of the merger effects from the empirical distribution of price changes across the control group hospitals.

Merger retrospectives typically employ a variant of the following model.

(1) $\ln p_i = X_i \beta + \delta_{h_i} + \alpha A_i + \phi A_i M_i + \varepsilon_i$

---

[26] See also; Town et al. (2006), who analyze the effect of hospital mergers on HMO premiums.

The log of price p_i charged to individual i is determined by characteristics X_i and a hospital fixed effect δ_{h_i}.[27] Dummy variable A_i takes a value of one if individual i enters hospital h_i after the merger is consummated. Similarly, M_i is a dummy variable for whether h_i is one of the merging hospitals. The coefficient ϕ of the interaction term $A_i M_i$ is the "difference in difference" estimate of interest, as it reports the post-merger price change of the merging hospitals relative to the control group.

The validity of this exercise depends on the properties of the error term ε_i. For example, the error terms of individuals who enter the same hospital, and who have the same insurer, are likely correlated when the price charged for each individual is determined by the same contract. In this case, estimation of equation (1) via ordinary least squares (OLS) leads to standard errors that are typically downwards biased (Moulton, 1990; Bertrand et al., 2004).

A simple example demonstrates this point. Suppose there are two hospitals, the merging hospital h_{merge} and a control hospital h_{ctrl}. For the merging hospital, the log price change from the pre- to post-merger time period is ϕ_{merge}. Similarly, let ϕ_{ctrl} be the price change for the control hospital. Suppose one can perfectly observe these price changes. One might (erroneously) conclude that if $\phi_{merge} \neq \phi_{ctrl}$, the merger has an impact on price. Random variation across hospitals, however, will generally lead to some difference between ϕ_{merge} and ϕ_{ctrl}. Let $\phi_{merge} = \theta + \omega_{merge}$, where θ is the effect of the merger and ω_{merge} is i.i.d $N(0,\sigma^2)$. Let $\phi_{ctrl} = \omega_{ctrl}$, where ω_{ctrl} is also i.i.d $N(0,\sigma^2)$. Under this specification, the probability that $\phi_{merge} \neq \phi_{ctrl}$ is one. Thus, if one ignores the impact of random variation in hospital prices, one will always conclude that the merger has an effect. The standard error of the difference in each hospital's price change is $\sqrt{2\sigma^2}$, rather than zero. With only two hospitals, however, one cannot estimate the degree of inter-hospital heterogeneity σ^2. As such, in this simple example it is impossible to test whether the merger has an impact on price.

---

[27] In our empirical analysis, we separately estimate the post-merger price change for each health insurer.

Suppose there are n hospitals, where n is at least three. As before, assume that one can perfectly observe the price change ϕ_h for each hospital. It now becomes possible to test whether the merger has an impact by estimating the following model.

(2) $\qquad \phi_h = Z_h \gamma + \theta M_h + \omega_h$

Hospital characteristics Z_h control for factors that explain variation in each hospital's post-merger price change. As before, M_h is a dummy variable for the merging hospitals, so that θ represents the merging parties' price change relative to the control group. Assuming that ω_h is i.i.d Normally distributed, equation (2) satisfies the classic Normal regression model. This implies that unbiased standard errors are obtained by estimating the model via OLS. Note that the number of observations in equation (2) is equal to the number of hospitals, not the number of patients. The obtained estimates will generally be imprecise when the number of control hospitals is small.

In practice, each hospital's post-merger price change ϕ_h is not directly observed, but must be estimated. One possibility is the following adaptation of equation (1):

(3) $\qquad \ln p_i = X_i \beta + \delta_{h_i} + \sum_h \phi_h A_i 1_{h_i = h} + \varepsilon_i$

This specification is inappropriate for analyzing hospital mergers due to the use of contractual arrangements. Contracts between a hospital and insurance companies may not expire immediately upon consummation of the merger. A post-merger price change might not be implemented until the current contract ends.

To address this issue, we generalize equation (3) by including a set of fixed effects that vary by quarter of year t for each hospital h.

(4) $\qquad \ln p_i = X_i \beta + \delta_{h_i, t_i} + \varepsilon_i$

Each hospital's post-merger price increase ϕ_h is calculated as follows. We allow for a one-year transition period during which old contracts expire and new ones are negotiated. Since the Sutter-Summit transaction was consummated in the final days of 1999, we do not use data from

January to December 2000 when estimating the post-merger price change. Rather, we define the post-merger period as January to December 2001.[28] Similarly, the pre-merger period is January to December 1999. For each hospital, the post-merger price change ϕ_h is calculated as the difference between the average estimate of $\delta_{h,t}$ across the four quarters in 2001 and the average across the four quarters in 1999. These estimates are then used as the dependent variable in equation (2).[29]

To summarize, we measure the post-merger price change at Summit and Alta Bates relative to the price change for a set of control group hospitals using a two-stage estimation method. In the first stage, we estimate equation (4) to obtain a measure of each hospital's price in both the pre- and post-merger periods. The post-merger price change for Summit, Alta Bates, and the control group hospitals is calculated from these price measures, which are then used as the dependent variable in equation (2). This produces an estimate of the difference in the post-merger price change between the merging parties and the control group hospitals. Importantly, this method estimates the standard error of the merger effect based on the empirical distribution of price changes across the control group hospitals. This allows us to determine whether the price change for the merging parties is sufficiently unusual that it can be reasonably attributed to the Sutter-Summit transaction.

IV. Data

Our analysis relies on commercial claims data provided by Summit, Alta Bates, and three large health insurers. The data provided by Summit and Alta Bates contains admissions records for a larger number of health insurers, but only for admissions at these two hospitals. In contrast,

---

[28] One insurer in our data did not negotiate a new contract until 2002. For this insurer we analyze the price change between 1999 and 2002.

[29] The construction of each hospital's post-merger price change leads to some estimation error due to random sampling, which potentially creates a heteroskedastic error term in equation (2). This has little impact on our analysis, however, since we focus on large hospitals where each post-merger price change is estimated quite precisely relative to the variance of the error term.

the health insurer data covers only three health insurers, but contains admissions to any hospital in California. We use this data to compare Summit and Alta Bates' post-merger price change to the price change for a control group of comparable hospitals that did not undergo merger.

We focus on acute inpatient hospital care. As explained in section II, this set of services has traditionally been the product market employed in hospital mergers, as only relatively poor substitutes exist outside of hospitals.

The dependent variable in our analysis is the price charged for each hospital admission. This is defined as total payments for hospital services across all sources, including insurance companies and payments made by those receiving care (e.g., co-payments). For a small number of claims, the average payment per admission day is implausibly small due to incomplete records, non-covered benefits, and other such problems. We therefore restrict the dataset to claims where the average payment per day is at least $200.

As explained in the previous section, we employ the regression framework specified in equation (4), where the log of total payments is determined by the control variables listed in the following table. Sets of dummy variables are used to control for the discrete (categorical) variables, while fourth order polynomials are used for the continuous variables. This allows for a high degree of flexibility in the model specification.

Patient-Level Controls

Admission Length	Dummy variables are used for each admission length up to 30 days, which comprises the vast majority of claims. A fourth order polynomial is employed for longer admission lengths.
Diagnosis	Admissions widely vary with regard to the complexity of care involved. Depending on which variable is reported for a given dataset, we control for each claim's DRG or for its ICD9 primary diagnosis.[30] We do so using a set of dummy variables for each DRG or ICD9 category.[31]
Cost Categories	Some datasets report the cost category to which each admission belongs (e.g., NICU, Cardiovascular Surgery, etc.). When available, we employ a set of dummy variables for each cost category.
Plan Type	For commercial claims, we use dummy variables for each type of insurance plan (e.g., HMO, PPO, etc.)
Sex	A dummy variable for each patient's gender is employed.
Age	The patient's age at the time of admission is controlled for using a fourth order polynomial. A dummy variable for whether the patient is a newborn is also included.

These variables explain cross-sectional (inter-patient) differences in hospital payments. However, they do not control for overall price changes at each hospital. Such changes are controlled for using a set of fixed effects that vary by hospital and quarter year. As explained in section III, these fixed effects comprise the basis of our analysis. Each dataset reports patient-level claims starting in 1997 or 1998, depending on the dataset, and continuing until 2001 or 2002.

When analyzing the datasets provided by the three insurance companies, we compare Summit and Alta Bates to other hospitals in California. To maintain similarity with the merging hospitals, we restrict attention to urban, non-government, general service hospitals with at least 200 beds (Source: American Hospital Association). Further, we remove hospitals that have

---

[30] As explained in Krishnan (2001), "DRGs are a set of case types established under the Medicare Prospective Payment System (PPS) identifying patients with similar conditions and processes of care."

[31] There are a very large number of ICD9 codes, making it impractical to employ fixed effects for each. However, ICD9 diagnoses are classified into a smaller number of categories. We employ fixed effects for each category.

recently been involved in a merger (Source: Irving Levin Associates), as well as other hospitals in the same metropolitan statistical area. Finally, to exclude hospitals with only sporadic admissions for a given payer, we restrict attention to those hospitals that admit one or more patients per week at least 95% of the time (for the particular payer being considered). These restrictions yield a relatively large set of hospitals, between 40 and 71 hospitals depending on the insurer.

Even within these relatively homogenous hospitals, some differences in observable characteristics remain. Therefore, when estimating equation (2) we control for several additional factors that potentially explain inter-hospital price variation. Note that we use these variables to explain variation in price growth between the pre- and post-merger periods, not inter-hospital differences in price levels (which are captured by the hospital specific fixed effects that are differenced out when calculating each hospital's post-merger price change ϕ_h).[32]

The control variables employed are listed in the following table. They are constructed using data for the year 1997, which is when the claims-level datasets described above first report patient admissions.

---

[32] Changes in these variables between the pre- and post-merger periods potentially explain each hospital's change in price. Controlling for this possibility is impractical (and unnecessary), however, since these characteristics undergo very little variation over time.

Hospital-Level Controls

Teaching Hospital A dummy variable for whether a hospital is a member of the Council of Teaching Hospitals of the Association of American Medical Colleges (Source: AHA).

Beds The total number of beds staffed for inpatient use (Source: AHA).

Case Mix The case mix index measures the resources needed to treat the mix of patients admitted to each hospital (Source: OSHPD).

For-profit Hospital A dummy variable for whether a hospital is a for-profit business (Source: AHA).

% Medicare The fraction of total admission days that correspond to Medicare patients (Source: OSHPD).

% Medicaid The fraction of total admission days that correspond to Medicaid patients (Source: OSHPD).

Southern California A dummy variable for whether a hospital is located in Southern California. Southern California is defined as the portion of the state south of (and including) the following counties: San Luis Obispo, Kern, and San Bernardino.

Notes: AHA=American Hospital Association, OSHPD=Office of Statewide Health Planning and Development.

The first three variables proxy for inter-hospital differences in costs and the range of services provided. A for-profit dummy variable is employed in response to the literature's concern that for- and non-profit hospitals have different objectives when setting price. The variables that control for a hospital's dependence on Medicare and Medicaid are included to control for cross-subsidization between these categories and commercial claims. For example, a cutback in Medicare and Medicaid reimbursements might induce hospitals to increase price for their commercial patients (Dranove and White, 1998). Lastly, since California is a large state we control for potential differences between the northern and the southern regions.

V.   Results

First, we estimate equation (4) using Summit and Alta Bates' internal admission records for five health insurers. In addition to the other control variables mentioned in section IV, separate sets of quarter-year fixed effects are estimated for each hospital and health insurance provider. These are the estimates of primary interest, since they report how each hospital's price changed after the merger.

The first two columns of Table 1 present the post-merger price change for each insurer.[33] While price increased at both hospitals for every insurer, the price increase is substantially larger at Summit. The price increase for Alta Bates ranges from 10.2% to 20.7%, depending on the insurer, compared to 29.0% to 72.0% at Summit. Columns 3 and 4 of Table 1 report the price difference between the two hospitals in both the pre- and post-merger periods. Pre-merger, Summit's price is substantially below Alta Bates' price for all five insurers. The difference ranges from 21.7% to 47.2%. Post-merger, prices at the two hospitals substantially converge. The magnitude of the price difference is less than 5% for three of the insurers, with Summit 8.9% to 13.8% lower priced for the other two insurers.

While informative, these results do not directly speak to whether the price at either hospital increased by more than it would have but for the merger. As discussed earlier, a control group of similar hospitals is required to distinguish a merger related price increase from price variation unrelated to the transaction. To address this issue, we estimate models (2) and (4) using claims data provided by three large health insurers. These datasets contain admission records for a large number of similar hospitals, allowing us to compare Summit and Alta Bates' post-merger price change to the empirical distribution of price changes for the control group.

Table 2 reports the results from this analysis, which employs the hospital control group detailed earlier in section IV. For all three insurers, Summit's post-merger price change is among the largest of any comparable hospital in California. Depending on the insurer, the Summit price increase is between the 95th and 99th percentile of the distribution of price changes across the control group hospitals. In contrast, Alta Bates' post-merger price change is quite typical, with many other hospitals having either smaller or larger price changes.

---

[33] To minimize concerns regarding confidentiality, we only report those results of direct interest to this paper.

Regression analysis confirms this conclusion. In the first specification, which employs only dummy variables for the merging hospitals, Summit's post-merger price change is 28.4% to 44.2% larger than the average price change for the control group, depending on the insurer. These estimates are all statistically significant at the 5% level. In contrast, Alta Bates' price change is never statistically different from the control group.

There is significant heterogeneity in the post-merger price change across the control group hospitals. Since some of this variation may be explained by each hospital's observable characteristics, Table 2 reports results from a second regression that controls for the hospital characteristics detailed in section IV. For Insurer 1, several of these variables are statistically significant. The additional controls are not individually (or jointly) significant for the other two insurers.

For all three insurers the inclusion of hospital characteristics has limited effect on the estimates of the merger's impact. Summit's price increase relative to the control group ranges from 23.2% to 50.4%, depending on the insurer. The estimates for Insurer 1 and Insurer 2 are statistically significant at the 5% level. The estimate for Insurer 3 is statistically significant only at the 10% level, with a p-value of .057. As before, the Alta Bates price increase is not statistically different from the control group for any of the insurers.

To summarize, our results indicate that the Sutter-Summit transaction led to a large price increase at Summit, but did not have a statistically significant impact on Alta Bates' price. As discussed earlier in section II, one explanation for this asymmetry is that as a large provider of hospital services to commercial patients, Alta Bates was a major constraint on Summit's price. Post-merger, the two hospitals internalized this constraint, leading to higher prices at Summit. In contrast, pre-merger Summit attracted relatively few commercial patients. To the extent that Alta Bates' pre-merger price was primarily constrained by other hospitals that, unlike Summit, attracted large numbers of commercial patients, one would not expect the Sutter-Summit transaction to substantially increase Alta Bates' price. Our results are consistent with this explanation.

A key assumption in our analysis is that, but for the merger, the price increase at Summit and Alta Bates would have been similar to the price change for the control group hospitals. The Sutter-Summit transaction is arguably not an exogenous source of variation. Unobserved variables that precipitated the merger might be correlated with other factors that could have caused Summit's price increase, potentially biasing our results.

Summit began the process of seeking potential purchasers in 1995, leading to merger negotiations that ultimately led to the Sutter-Summit transaction.[34] We indirectly test for endogeneity bias by exploiting the four-year lag between when Summit initially sought a partner and it was ultimately acquired in 1999. If the factors that caused Summit to search for a partner were correlated with unobservables that affected Summit's pricing, then one would expect its pre-merger pricing to differ from the control group hospitals.

We test this proposition by repeating our analysis using price changes from 1997-1999, rather than from 1999-2001. By doing so, we study whether Summit behaved unusually pre-merger, relative to the control group. If so, this would cast doubt on Summit's comparability to the control hospitals in the post-merger period. The results from this analysis are presented in Table 3. The 1997-1999 price change for both Summit and Alta Bates is very similar to, and statistically indistinguishable from, the control group hospitals. Thus, the unusually high post-merger price change at Summit cannot be explained by a similarly unusual price change in the period preceding the merger.

A related concern is that Summit may have increased price post-merger due to the financial difficulties it was experiencing at the time, rather than due to the merger itself. Summit's financial condition was sufficiently dire that the judge in the preliminary injunction trial concluded Summit was a "failing firm."[35] If hospitals in poor financial condition engage in different pricing behavior than other hospitals, then our results could potentially be biased. It is

---

[34] California v. Sutter Health System, 130 F. Supp. 2d at 1115 (N.D. California, 2001).

[35] California v. Sutter Health System, 130 F. Supp. 2d at 1137 (N.D. California, 2001).

important to note, however, that the deterioration of Summit's financial condition substantially preceded the Sutter-Summit transaction. A major reason for Summit's financial problems was the Balanced Budget Act of 1997, signed into law on August 5, 1997, which significantly reduced Summit's reimbursement for Medicare patients.[36] As detailed above, Summit's price change over the period 1997-1999 was similar to the price change for the control group hospitals. It seems unlikely that a 1997 change in Medicare reimbursement significantly affected Summit's price change for the period 1999-2001 when it had little apparent effect on Summit's price change for the period 1997-1999.

VI. Conclusion

This paper investigates whether the Sutter-Summit transaction affected inpatient hospital prices for commercial patients. Our results indicate that this merger led to a large price increase at Summit, but did not have a statistically significant impact on Alta Bates' price. One explanation for this asymmetry is that as a major provider of hospital services to commercial patients in the Oakland-Berkeley area, Alta Bates was a significant price constraint on Summit. However, Summit may have been less of a constraint on Alta Bates' price since Summit was a relatively minor provider of hospital services to commercial patients.

Prior to the transaction, Summit officials predicted that it "would give them more clout in negotiating with health insurers..."[37] Presumably, one of the benefits of increased bargaining power is the ability to charge higher prices. The large post-merger price increase found in this paper is therefore consistent with Summit's own pre-merger prediction.

Summit and Alta Bates were located in a large urban area with many other hospitals that offered a similar range of services. Based on patient flow data, one might conclude that consumers (and health insurance providers) could turn to many other hospitals for care. A

---

[36] California v. Sutter Health System, 130 F. Supp. 2d at 1115 (N.D. California, 2001).

[37] "Summit Medical to Join Sutter." *San Francisco Chronicle*, March 27, 1998.

central issue raised by the Sutter-Summit transaction was whether this patient flow indicated that travel costs were sufficiently low that the presence of other hospitals would prevent an anticompetitive price increase. Our results suggest they were an insufficient constraint.

Summit and Alta Bates were both non-profits, a characteristic that some researchers argue makes hospitals less likely to engage in a post-merger price increase. Our results demonstrate that non-profit hospitals may still raise price quite substantially after they merge. This suggests that mergers involving non-profit hospitals should perhaps attract as much antitrust scrutiny as other hospital mergers.

One should not infer too much from a case study of a single hospital merger. It may be inappropriate to generalize our results to other hospital mergers. Instead, our findings should be viewed as an incremental contribution to the growing body of evidence regarding the effectiveness of antitrust policy.

References

American Hospital Association. 1997. *AHA Guide to the Health Care Field.* Chicago, IL.

Bertrand, Marianne, Esther Duflo, and Sendhil Mullainathan. 2004. "How Much Should We Trust Differences-in-Differences Estimates?" *Quarterly Journal of Economics* 119(1):249-75.

Capps, Cory and David Dranove. 2004. "Hospital Consolidation and Negotiated PPO Prices." *Health Affairs* 23(2):175-81.

Capps, Corry, David Dranove, Shane Greenstein, and Mark Satterthwaite. 2001. "The Silent Majority Fallacy of the Elzinga-Hogarty Criteria: A Critique and New Approach to Analyzing Hospital Mergers." NBER Working Paper #8216.

Capps, Corry, David Dranove, and Mark Satterthwaite. 2003. "Competition and Market Power in Option Demand Markets." *RAND Journal of Economics* 34(4):737-63.

Conner, Robert A., Roger D. Feldman and Bryan E. Dowd. 1998. "The Effects of Market Concentration and Horizontal Mergers on Hospital Costs and Prices." *International Journal of the Economics of Business* 5(2):159-80.

Dranove, David and Richard Ludwick. 1999. "Competition and Pricing by Nonprofit Hospitals: A Reassessment of Lynk's Analysis." *Journal of Health Economics* 18(1):87-98.

Dranove, David and William D. White. 1998. "Medicaid-Dependent Hospitals and Their Patients: How Have They Fared?" *Health Services Research* 33(2):163-85.

Elzinga, Kenneth G. and Thomas F. Hogarty. 1973. "The Problem of Geographic Market Delineation in Antimerger Suits." *Antitrust Bulletin* 18(1): 45-81.

Elzinga, Kenneth G. and Thomas F. Hogarty. 1978. "The Problem of Geographic Market Definition Revisited: The Case of Coal." *Antitrust Bulletin* 23(1):1-18.

Gaynor, Martin and William B. Vogt. 1999. "Antitrust and Competition in Health Care Markets." NBER Working Paper #7112.

Gaynor, Martin and William B. Vogt. 2003. "Competition among Hospitals." *RAND Journal of Economics* 34(4):764-85.

Harrison, Teresa D. and Kristina M. Lybecker. 2005. "The Effect of the Nonprofit Motive on Hospital Competitive Behavior." *B.E. Journals in Economic Analysis and Policy: Contributions to Economic Analysis and Policy* 4(1):1-15.

Irving Levin Associates. Various years. *The Hospital Acquisition Report.* New Canaan, Ct.

Keeler, Emmett B. and Glenn Melnick and Jack Zwanziger. 1999. "The Changing Effects of Competition on Non-Profit and For-Profit Hospital Pricing Behavior." *Journal of Health Economics* 18(1): 69-86.

Krishnan, Ranjani. 2001. "Market Restructuring and Pricing in the Hospital Industry." *Journal of Health Economics* 20(2):213-37.

Lynk, William J. 1995. "Nonprofit Hospital Mergers and the Exercise of Market Power." *Journal of Law and Economics* 38(2):437-61.

Lynk, William J. and Lynette R. Neumann. 1999. "Price and Profit." *Journal of Health Economics* 18(1):99-116.

Moulton, Brent R. 1990. "An Illustration of a Pitfall in Estimating the Effects of Aggregate Variables on Micro Units." *Review of Economics and Statistics* 72(2):334-38.

Newhouse, Joseph P. 1970. "Toward a Theory of Nonprofit Institutions: An Economic Model of a Hospital." *American Economic Review* 60(1):64-74.

Sacher, Seth and Louis Silvia. 1998. "Antitrust Issues in Defining the Product Market for Hospital Services." *International Journal of the Economics of Business* 5(2):181-202.

Simpson, John and Richard Shin. 1998. "Do Nonprofit Hospitals Exercise Market Power?" *International Journal of the Economics of Business* 5(2):141-57.

Taylor, Christopher T. and Daniel S. Hosken. 2007. "The Economic Effects of the Marathon-Ashland Joint Venture: The Importance of Industry Supply Shocks and Vertical Market Structure." *Journal of Industrial Economics* 55(3):419-51.

Town, Robert and Gregory Vistnes. 2001. "Hospital Competition in HMO Networks." *Journal of Health Economics* 20(5):733-53.

Town, Robert, Douglas Wholey, Roger Feldman, and Lawton R. Burns. 2006. "The Welfare Consequences of Hospital Mergers." NBER Working Paper #12244.

Vita, Michael G. and Seth Sacher. 2001. "The Competitive Effects of Not-for-Profit Hospital Mergers: A Case Study." *Journal of Industrial Economics* 49(1):63-84.

Werden, Gregory J. 1981. "On the Use and Misuse of Shipments Data in Defining Geographic Markets." *Antitrust Bulletin* 26(4):719-37.

Werden, Gregory J. 1990. "The Limited Relevance of Patient Migration Data in Market Delineation for Hospital Merger Cases." *Journal of Health Economics* 8(4):363-76.

Table 1: Post-merger Price Change

	Post-merger Price Change		Summit - Alta Bates Price Gap	
	Summit	Alta Bates	Pre-merger	Post-merger
Insurer 1	**42.1%**	**19.8%**	**-21.7%**	**0.6%**
	(1.9%)	(1.7%)	(1.9%)	(1.7%)
Insurer 2	**44.7%**	**12.0%**	**-37.7%**	**-5.0%**
	(2.5%)	(2.1%)	(2.6%)	(2.0%)
Insurer 3	**72.0%**	**20.7%**	**-47.2%**	**4.0%**
	(2.2%)	(3.2%)	(3.0%)	(2.5%)
Insurer 4	**31.9%**	**11.5%**	**-34.1%**	**-13.8%**
	(3.5%)	(4.4%)	(4.6%)	(3.5%)
Insurer 5	**29.0%**	**10.2%**	**-27.7%**	**-8.9%**
	(4.7%)	(8.6%)	(7.9%)	(5.8%)

Data Source: Admission records provided by Summit and Alta Bates.

Notes: N=24,281, R^2=.84, and RMSE=.42. The dependent variable is the log price of each admission. The model controls for admission length, DRG, plan type, sex, and age (see text for details). Heteroskedastic robust standard errors are reported in parentheses.

Table 2: Post-merger Price Change Relative to the Control Group

	Insurer 1			Insurer 2			Insurer 3		
Post-merger Price Change Percentile Rank:									
Summit	99%			96%			95%		
Alta Bates	89%			65%			23%		
Model Specification 1:									
	Est	**SE**		**Est**	**SE**		**Est**	**SE**	
Intercept	16.1%	1.1%		15.8%	1.5%		29.5%	3.4%	
Summit	*28.7%*	*9.1%*	***	*28.4%*	*10.7%*	**	*44.2%*	*21.4%*	**
Alta Bates	*14.1%*	*9.1%*		*0.9%*	*10.7%*		*-12.6%*	*21.4%*	
R^2:	0.15			0.13			0.11		
RMSE:	0.09			0.11			0.21		
Model Specification 2:									
	Est	**SE**		**Est**	**SE**		**Est**	**SE**	
Intercept	-11.7%	11.9%		7.7%	22.3%		-9.6%	57.1%	
Summit	*23.2%*	*8.7%*	***	*24.8%*	*12.1%*	**	*50.4%*	*25.4%*	*
Alta Bates	*7.1%*	*9.0%*		*-8.7%*	*12.5%*		*-2.4%*	*26.4%*	
Teaching Hospital	-8.7%	4.7%	*	-9.0%	7.8%		-3.0%	17.3%	
Southern CA	-4.6%	2.4%	*	-1.2%	3.7%		6.6%	9.2%	
Beds / 100	1.9%	1.2%		3.4%	2.1%		-2.8%	5.0%	
Case Mix	15.9%	6.2%	**	1.3%	11.3%		30.1%	28.2%	
% Medicare	3.0%	11.1%		-7.8%	20.2%		-2.3%	45.6%	
% Medicaid	-5.8%	9.6%		-2.1%	20.1%		-6.2%	46.3%	
For-profit Hospital	0.0%	2.9%		-5.2%	5.4%		-15.6%	11.4%	
R^2:	0.37			0.22			0.20		
RMSE:	0.08			0.11			0.22		

Data Source: Admission records provided by three health insurers.

Notes: For each insurer, the dependent variable is the log price change at each hospital between the pre- and post-merger period. These price changes are calculated from a set of hospital * time fixed effects estimated using regression model (4). This first stage regression controls for admission length, ICD9 primary diagnosis, cost category (when available), plan type, sex, and age (see text for details). Statistics from the first stage regressions are: Insurer 1 (R^2=.82, RMSE=.42), Insurer 2 (R^2=.85, RMSE=.36), and Insurer 3 (R^2=.84, RMSE=.40). Significance levels are defined as *=10%, **=5%, and ***=1%.

Table 3: Pre-merger Price Change Relative to the Control Group

	Insurer 1		Insurer 2		Insurer 3	
Pre-merger Price Change Percentile Rank:						
Summit	66%		47%		43%	
Alta Bates	65%		67%		53%	
Model Specification 1:						
	Est	**SE**	**Est**	**SE**	**Est**	**SE**
Intercept	6.1%	1.2%	4.7%	1.8%	2.0%	1.4%
Summit	*1.9%*	*10.1%*	*0.2%*	*12.7%*	*-1.1%*	*8.4%*
Alta Bates	*1.4%*	*10.1%*	*3.6%*	*12.7%*	*-0.1%*	*8.4%*
R^2:	0.00		0.00		0.00	
RMSE:	0.10		0.12		0.08	
Model Specification 2:						
	Est	**SE**	**Est**	**SE**	**Est**	**SE**
Intercept	-1.9%	13.4%	42.9%	26.5%	-8.7%	21.1%
Summit	*-5.1%*	*9.9%*	*1.6%*	*14.4%*	*0.3%*	*9.4%*
Alta Bates	*-7.4%*	*10.1%*	*7.7%*	*14.9%*	*-2.2%*	*9.8%*
Teaching Hospital	-5.6%	5.3%	11.8%	9.3%	-10.2%	6.4%
Southern CA	-8.6%	2.7% ***	-6.1%	4.4%	-0.6%	3.4%
Beds / 100	1.1%	1.4%	-2.3%	2.5%	0.4%	1.8%
Case Mix	9.5%	7.0%	-12.6%	13.5%	11.9%	10.4%
% Medicare	-4.6%	12.5%	-7.8%	24.0%	-17.8%	16.9%
% Medicaid	-10.4%	10.9%	-29.1%	24.0%	-8.6%	17.1%
For-profit Hospital	-2.4%	3.2%	1.8%	6.5%	-1.3%	4.2%
R^2:	0.24		0.11		0.21	
RMSE:	0.09		0.13		0.08	

Data Source: Admission records provided by three health insurers.

Notes: For each insurer, the dependent variable is the log price change at each hospital between 1997 and 1999. These price changes are calculated from a set of hospital * time fixed effects estimated using regression model (4). This first stage regression controls for admission length, ICD9 primary diagnosis, cost category (when available), plan type, sex, and age (see text for details). Statistics from the first stage regressions are: Insurer 1 (R^2=.82, RMSE=.42), Insurer 2 (R^2=.85, RMSE=.36), and Insurer 3 (R^2=.84, RMSE=.40). Significance levels are defined as *=10%, **=5%, and ***=1%.